SIRTFOOD DIET FOR BEGINNERS:

A complete guide for beginners to activate the Skinny gene and lose weight. With over 150 Sirtfood recipes to burn fat in an intelligent way for your body and mind.

Table of Contents

Introduction

The most recent diet rinse which has the world raving about it follows a scientific way to deal with fight weight gain.

The diet advances on the utilization of 'Sirtfoods', which are some uncommon nourishment which work by enacting certain protein chains in the body, known as sirtuins. According to science, these cancer prevention agent operators go about as protectants that help hinder maturing, support digestion and control the body's irritation, thus helping in fat loss.

Studies have likewise discovered that the sirtfood diet can assist individuals with losing as much as seven pounds (3 kilos) in less than seven days' time.

The diet, however viewed as a craze, focuses on keeping up a prohibitive weight loss methodology multi week. While the initial three days makes you limit your calorie admission to 1000kcal (expending three sirt nourishment green squeezes and having a dinner). The rest of the days, you are permitted to expand your calorie admission to 1500kcal and have two suppers per day (alongside two sirtfood juices). Post this, the support stage prescribes you to eat up to three adjusted nourishments rich in sirtuin, combined with a successful workout methodology to get thinner, making it even more maintainable.

Since it is fairly prohibitive in nature, many remain careful about the diet plan working over the long haul. The diet confines your calorie allow and can void you of other required supplements, in this way, it's anything but a long haul, economical diet plan for weight loss.

1. Discontinuous fasting – One of the most well-known diet which cycles around a time of fasting and eating. The most widely recognized is 16:8 strategies where you eat for 8 hours and the rest 16 hours is fasting period where you don't eat anything or you can have water if parched. Medical advantages incorporate are decreased aggravation, diminishes muscle to fat ratio stores, battle against malignant growth, lessens cholesterol level, diabetes.

2. Paleo diet – A pattern which centers around nutrition classes, for example, crisp foods grown from the ground, seeds and nuts, lean meat, fish that is wealthy in omega 3, natural oil.

3. Vegetarian lifestyle – A lifestyle wherein individuals keep away from every one of the items that are gotten from a creature like meat, eggs and all the dairy items however can expend a wide range of organic products, vegetables, grains, vegetables, nuts and seeds. They even limit themselves from gaining any family unit or individual stuff that originates from creatures. The advantages of following such a lifestyle are decreased cardiovascular hazard, diabetes, weight loss and so forth.

4. Without gluten diet – An eating design where you maintain a strategic distance from any nourishment thing that has gluten in it, for example, wheat, rye, grain however separated from this you can appreciate crisp organic product, vegetables, fish, all the dairy item, seeds, nuts, flours which has no gluten present in it. Diminishes muscle to fat ratio stores, swelling, obstruction, improves insusceptible arrangement of the body.

5. Run diet – The Dietary Approaches to Stop Hypertension (DASH) diet is a low sodium, low fat diet. It is wealthy in foods grown from the ground, which guarantees a significant inventory of minerals and nutrients. A scramble diet centers on entire nourishments and rejects all types of handled nourishment.

Nourishments high in fat have been connected to poor, divided rest. Fat triggers the stomach related procedures and causes a development of stomach acids, which while resting can cause distress. However, before starting a new diet to lose weight, our advice is to have a specialist follow you because psychophysical well-being also passes through a correct and tailor-made diet.

Chapter 1.   Sirt Diet Story

The Sirt food diet and Lorraine Pascale:

Lorraine Pascale is probably the world's most well-known and well-praised chef and food enthusiast. She belongs to the United Kingdom, the same country in which the Sirt food diet was first introduced. She is known as a successful supermodel when Lorraine was sixteen years old. She took care of her chronically ill mother for many years, and it was the time when she found the importance of some particular foods in the nourishment of chronically ill patients. This turned her interests in entirely different directions. She started taking an interest in cooking, and in no time, she was recognized as the most well-known and widely praised chef of the world. She has written many books on diet and foods. Over one million copies of her books were sold solely in UK, and this a huge success indeed. She is a TV host, and her shows are aired in more than 70 countries globally. The ratings of her shows are insane, and she is the most-watched chef globally.

The praise of the Sirt food diet from the guru herself was a significant breakthrough in the popularity of this dieting regime. She mentioned that the Sirt food diet is the best-known diet for her with thousands of benefits. She considers herself as the biggest fan of the Sirt food diet, which is enough with respect to the Sirt food diet. She mentioned that the Sirt food diet was a breakthrough in achieving the best shape of her life; even this person is a supermodel herself. So notably, these statements from the Lorraine Pascale are enough to establish the health benefits of the Sirt food diet.

David Haye and the Sirt food diet:

He is one of the most dynamic boxers in history. He belongs to the UK, and he has won many titles of boxing championships. He has fought for two different weight classes in the same year and won both titles as the world's champion, thanks to the Sirt food diet and his fantastic training. David Haye is a vegan who loves vegan foods. He also holds a company that makes vegan protein powders. The number one problem of different fat loss diets is the issue related to vegan followers. Most of the ordinary fat loss diets involve a high protein diet coming from the animal source, which is, of course, big trouble for vegan lovers. Some fat loss diets are also designed for vegans, and these diets don't have any space for the meat lovers. So this cross completion between vegan and non-vegan interest causes many issues for both categories. The Sirt food diet is unique in this regard. It contains a great variety of vegan foods as well as a perfect space for meat lovers. The diet can be modified according to personal interest, and it is a win-win situation for both. The consumer just has to stick with the basic principles of the Sirt food diet, which are very simple to follow.

This perfect diet for vegans provided significant benefits to vegan boxer David Haye during his competitions. He mentioned that the Sirt food diet provided him the most significant benefits of his career by refueling his body with a lot of energy and an easy ladder to climb up on higher weight class and winning the title against a competitor who contained 9-inch height and 45 kg weight benefit on David Haye. But his amazing skills and high energy provided by the Sirt food diet provided him with the new world heavyweight title. It is enough to describe the benefits of the Sirt food diet.

Jodie Kidd and the Sirt food diet:

Jodie Kidd is a British celebrity and supermodel who started her modeling career in just 16 years of age. At that time, she was 6 feet and 1 inch tall, with just 48 kg of body weight. Her slender physique was very famous among girls, and it was also reported that some girls turned anorexic after following her beauty standards. She took eight months from her modeling career and started eating a more caloric diet, so; size 14 was achieved in dresses worn by Jodie Kidd in those eight months. She was slender, and her most significant issue was putting on some weight rather than losing it. So, it was much different than introduced by nearly all fat loss diets. She has to put some weight while keeping the total body fat percentage low and increasing the lean muscle mass. It is not less than a fat loss challenge, and physique like Jodie Kidd had, it was even more challenging to achieve that goal. She has made multiple transformations over the course of years. She is not only a supermodel but also a fast car racer and a television host. When asked from Jodie about her perfect shape and glowing skin, she said that all credits belong to the Sirt food diet. Interestingly, the Sirt food diet was thought of as a principle fat loss diet, but Jodie used this diet to put lean muscle mass on her making her more curvaceous and healthy-looking.

Jodie said that the Sirt food diet was a game-changer for her. She followed that regime and got the best shape of her life. It was hard to put weight on her lean body, but the Sirt food diet helped her to achieve her fitness goals. She mentioned that the Sirt food diet is the key behind her good looks. These statements in favor of the Sirt food diet made this diet even more popular among the fans of Jodie, and thousands of people started using this dieting regime.

James Haskell and the Sirt food diet:

James Haskell is a former professional rugby player who played for many years as a leading rugby star from the national rugby team of the UK. He was a fantastic rugby player in both under 16 and under 18 categories. James also played as a national rugby player from Wales and Ireland. He has one of the most successful careers in rugby. James Haskell is known for his incredible athletic energy and buffed physique. He has excellent lean muscle mass on his well-ripped body and a very low-fat percentage. James has maintained his physique for years keeping the right track on his diet and eating habits. His career of rugby is charming, and now he has a high motivation to compete as a pro-MMA fighter. He will compete in the heavyweight class in May 2020 and has firm hopes about a charming career in MMA as well. James Haskell has used the Sirt food diet to keep up his body according to the standards of the heavyweight class. His statement about the Sirt food diet is very famous as he claimed that the most excellent performances of his career in the 2015 rugby world cup were due to the Sirt food diet. He trained hard and smart by keeping the Sirt food diet on the table, and this leads to incredible energy levels in his body. This statement made the Sirt food diet extremely famous among his fans as well as among his competitors, and thousands of people have followed this diet plan to achieve the best in their lives.

Sir Ben Ainslie and the Sirt food diet:

Sir Ben Ainslie is the best sailor among the history of Great Britain. He is a British national who competed in many Olympic Games and won many titles to his names. He was a sailor when he was eight years old, and he competed internationally in japan at the age of twelve. In 1196 he won the first Olympic gold medal in sailing. The unique capabilities of Sir Ben Ainslie are scarce, and Ben holds medals in five different categories of sailing sports. He is one of three athletes worldwide historically who achieved this rank. Moreover, Ben is the second-best Olympic sailor who holds four gold medals in sailing sports. He is a well-known athlete of British history and praised by millions of fans. The statements of Sir Ben Ainslie about the Sirt food diet are very supportive, and Ben mentioned the Sirt food diet as the vital force behind his successful career. He said that the Sirt food diet helped him achieving the best shape of his life and the best performances of his career because of the fantastic energy and focused mind. His performances in the British-American cup are the most golden memories of his career, and he claims that the Sirt food diet helped him achieve his goals in perfection.

Adele and the Sirt food diet:

Last but not least, Adele and the Sirt food diet is probably the most fantastic story of 2020 in context to physical transformations. Adele belongs to the UK, and she has won the best singer awards throughout her career. She is no doubt one of the loveliest voices in English pop history. She has amazing vocals and a very charming personality. Adele is one of those celebrities who have struggled a lot to achieve a lean physique, but it was never easy for her before the Sirt food diet. She was chubby and got plenty of extra pounds on her body. She was quite happy with her outlook, but she is also aware of the health risks associated with high body fat percentages. Adele has reportedly lost nearly 40 pounds of extra fat from her body within a few months of following the Sirt food diet. This diet plan was also popular among many other celebrities, but the transformation shown by

Adele created an incredible hype of the Sirt food diet. She now has the best shape of her life and a fantastic body, which is much leaner and healthier than before. Adele is very vocal about the health benefits of the Sirt food diet, and because of her vast transformation, the Sirt food diet is known as "The Adele Diet."

So, these statements are enough to show the benefits associated with the Sirt food diet, and when used properly, the Sirt food diet can be a great precursor behind the success of your life-changing achievements.

Chapter 2.   How the Sirt Diet Works

First Phase: Drastic Calories Reduction

First Phase: First 3 days of the week

Monday: 3 green juices

- Breakfast: water + tea or espresso + a cup of green juice;

- Lunch: green juice

- Snack: a square of dark chocolate;

- Dinner: Sirt meal

- After dinner: a square of dark chocolate.

Drink the juices at three distinct times of the day (for example, in the morning as soon as you wake up, mid-morning and mid-afternoon) and choose the normal or vegan dish: pan-fried oriental prawns with buckwheat spaghetti or miso and tofu with sesame glaze and sautéed vegetables (vegan dish)

Tuesday: 3 green juices

- Breakfast: water + tea or espresso + a cup of green juice

- Lunch: 2 green juices before dinner;

- Snack: a square of dark chocolate;

- Dinner: Sirt meal

- After dinner: a square of dark chocolate.

Welcome to day 2 of the Sirt Food Diet. The formula is identical to that of the first day, and the only thing that changes is the solid meal. Today you will also have dark chocolate, and the same goes for tomorrow. This food is so wonderful that we don't need an excuse to eat it.

To earn the title of a "Sirt food", chocolate must be at least 85 percent cocoa. And even among the various types of chocolate with this percentage, not all of them are the same. Often this product is treated with an alkalizing agent (this is the so-called "Dutch process") to reduce its acidity and give it a darker color. Unfortunately, this process greatly reduces the flavonoids activating sirtuins, compromising their health benefits.

On the second day, you will intake 3 green Sirt juices and one solid meal (normal or vegan).

Wednesday: 3 green juices

- Breakfast: water + tea or espresso + a cup of green juice

- Lunch: 2 green juices before dinner;

- Snack: a square of dark chocolate;

- Dinner: Sirt meal

- After dinner: a square of dark chocolate.

You are now on the third day, and even if the format is once again identical to that of days 1 and 2, so the time has come to flavor everything with a fundamental ingredient. For thousands of years, chili has been a fundamental element of the gastronomic experiences of the whole world. This is the last day you will consume three green juices a day; tomorrow, you will switch to two. We, therefore, take this opportunity to browse other drinks that you can have during the Diet.

As for the effects on health, we have already seen that its spiciness is perfect for activating sirtuins and stimulating the metabolism. The applications of chili are endless, and therefore represent an easy way to consume Sirt food regularly.

On the third day, you will intake 3 green Sirt juices and 1 one solid meal (normal or vegan, see below).

Thursday: 3 green juices

- Breakfast: water + tea or espresso + a cup of green juice;

- Lunch: Sirt food;

- Snack: 1 green juice before dinner

- Dinner: Sirt food

The fourth day of the Sirt Food Diet has arrived, and you are halfway through your journey to a leaner and healthier body. The big change from the last three days is that you will only drink two juices instead of three and that you will have two solid meals instead of one. This means that on the fourth day and the upcoming ones, you will have two green juices and 2 solid meals, all delicious and rich in Sirt foods. The inclusion of Medjool dates in a list of foods that promote weight loss and good health may seem surprising. Especially when you think they contain 66 percent sugar.

On the fourth day, you will intake: 2 green Sirt juices, 2 solid meals (normal or vegan)

Friday: 2 green juices

- Breakfast: water + tea or espresso + a cup of green juice

- Lunch: Sirt food

- Snack: a green juice before dinner;

- Dinner: Sirt food

You have reached the fifth day, and the time has come to add fruits. Due to its high sugar content, fruits have been the subject of bad publicity. This does not apply to berries. Strawberries have a very low sugar content: one teaspoon per 100 grams. They also have an excellent effect on how the body processes simple sugars.

On the fifth day, you will intake 2 green Sirt juices and 2 solid meals (normal or vegan).

Saturday: 2 green juices

- Breakfast: water + tea or espresso + a cup of green juice

- Lunch: Sirt food

- Snack: a green juice before dinner;

- Dinner: Sirt food

There are no Sirt foods better than olive oil and red wine. Virgin olive oil is obtained from the fruit only by mechanical means, in conditions that do not deteriorate it, so that you can be sure of its quality and polyphenol content. "Extra virgin" oil is that of the first pressing ("virgin" is the result of the second) and therefore has more flavor and better quality: this is what we strongly recommend you to use when cooking.

No Sirt menu would be complete without red wine, one of the cornerstones of the Diet. It contains the activators of resveratrol and piceatannol sirtuins, which probably explain the longevity and slenderness associated with the traditional French way of life, and which are at the origin of the enthusiasm unleashed by Sirt foods.

On the sixth day, you will assume 2 green Sirt juices and 2 solid meals (normal or vegan).

Drink the juices at different times of the day (for example, the first in the morning as soon as you wake up or in the middle of the morning, the second in the middle of the afternoon) and choose the normal or vegan dishes: Super Sirt salad and grilled beef fillet with red wine sauce, onion rings, curly garlic kale and roasted potatoes with aromatic herbs or

Super lentil Sirt salad (vegan dish) and mole sauce of red beans with roasted potato (vegan dish).

Sunday: 2 green juices

- Breakfast: a bowl of Sirt Muesli + a cup of green juice

- Lunch: Sirt food

- Snack: a cup of green juice;

- Dinner: Sirt food

The seventh day is the last of phase 1 of the Diet. Instead of considering it as an end, see it as a beginning, because you are about to embark on a new life, in which Sirt foods will play a central role in your nutrition. Today's menu is a perfect example of how easy it is to integrate them in abundance into your Daily Diet. Just take your favorite dishes, and, with a pinch of creativity, you will turn them into a Sirt banquet.

On the seventh day, you will assume 2 green Sirt juices; 2 solid meals (normal or vegan).

Drink the juices at different times of the day (for example the first in the morning as soon as you wake up or in the middle of the morning, the second in the middle of the afternoon) and choose the normal or vegan dishes: Sirt omelet Sirt and baked chicken breast, walnut and parsley pesto and red onion salad or Waldron salad (vegan dish) and baked eggplant wedges together with walnut and parsley pesto and tomato salad (vegan dish).

During the second phase, there are no calorie restrictions but indications on which Sirt foods must be eaten to consolidate weight loss and not run the risk of getting the lost kilograms back.

Second Phase: Maintenance

Congratulations! You have finished the first "hardcore" week. The second phase is easier and is the actual incorporation of sirtuin-filled food selections to your everyday Diet or meals. You can call this the "maintenance stage."

By doing so, your body will undergo the fat-burning stage and muscle gain plus a boost on your immune system and overall health.

For this phase, you can now have 3 balanced Sirt food-filled meals each day plus 1 green juice a day.

There is no "dieting," but more on choosing healthier alternatives with adding Sirt food in each meal as much as possible.

I will be providing some recipes for tasty dishes with Sirt food inclusion to give you further an idea of how exciting and healthy this diet journey is.

Now you move back up to a regular calorie intake with the aim to keep your weight loss steady and your Sirt food intake high. You should have experienced some degree of weight loss by now, but you should also feel trimmer and re-invigorated.

Phase 2 lasts for 14 days. During this time, you eat 3 sirt food rich meals, 1 sirt food green juice, and up to 2 optional Sirt food bite snacks. Strict calorie-counting is actively discouraged – if you follow the recommendations and eat balanced meals of reasonable portions, you shouldn't feel hungry or be consuming too much.

You should consume the same beverages you were drinking in phase 1, with the slight chance that you are welcome to enjoy the occasional glass of red wine (don't drink more than 3 per week).

Chapter 3.   Description: Skinny Gene

Switch on your Skinny Genes is not a diet. It is a way of eating for life. It is an eating plan where you can indulge in wine, coffee and chocolate and other delicious food, every day. It's a way of eating where you can have balanced indulgence.

For many of us indulgence is not a word that we associate with weight loss. Weight loss is all about deprivation and missing out. It's about "being on a diet" and, usually, those diets work. Until you stop the diet or fall off the wagon or life gets in the way. Suddenly those kilos that you struggled so hard to get rid of by being good are right back there on your belly, your hips, your chin, exactly where you don't want them to be.

Switch on your Skinny Genes is a different way of looking at the way you eat. When you eat Skinny Genes style you are not on a diet. You are learning a way of eating that you can maintain for life, without the need to be good. And you have permission (in fact you are encouraged) to drink red wine and eat dark chocolate, forbidden foods in any usual weight loss plan.

Switch on your Skinny Genes is an eating plan that leaves you feeling full and satisfied, both in your body and your mind. It is a backed-by-science eating plan that turns on your fat burning cells and turns off hunger signals.

It sounds too good to be true, doesn't it? But right now, you are being introduced to the latest research that explains that particular foods, including wine, chocolate and coffee, are essential for ramping up your body's fat-burning engine, turning down your hunger switch and giving your cells energy and vitality.

Can you imagine looking, feeling and being better, just by changing what you eat? Switch on your Skinny Genes is not about deprivation. It is about eating real food to get real and permanent results.

Switch on Your Skinny Genes is all about

- Food that turns on your skinny genes

- Food that is delicious and varied

- Food that is nourishing

- Food that you can share with your family and friends

- Food that allows you to live your life without being "on a diet"

- Food that is plentiful

- Food that is filling

- Food that will not break the budget

You will learn that food is not the enemy. Imagine how easy your life will be when you embrace food as your friend, when you and the food you eat will enjoy a more satisfying relationship. You will oversee the way you eat. Hunger and cravings will no longer control you.

You will transform your health for the better. You will look and feel younger. You will maintain consistent energy levels all day. Your sleep will improve. And, if you continue to embrace the principles of Switch on your Skinny Genes, the benefits will be long-term.

This eating plan is all about eating quality, real, whole, nutrient-dense, readily available food in amounts that satisfy hunger and maintain consistent energy levels. It will challenge the way that you've been taught to look at nutrition.

Switch on your Skinny Genes is not about calorie counting or exhausting yourself with excessive exercise.

Switch on your Skinny Genes is about learning how you can eat well to improve your health and still enjoy food that is delicious and satisfying without going hungry or feeling that you are missing out.

Chapter 4.   How to Activate the Skinny Gene

The study proposed that the weight-control advantages of sirt foods occur in part from the polyphenol-antioxidant resveratrol revitalizing your skinny gene with a standard sirt food diet plan and this is confirmed by

Taking foods in the plan that are nutritious

Acute calorie restriction just 1,000 calories daily for the phase one stage "first three days" and 1,500 daily for the rest of the week. And most of those calories should be obtained from the juice.

As you already know, restricting calories is the most dependable strategy for shedding weight. And for it is worthy, research from Finland's Helsinki University discovered that low-calorie foods might naturally improve sirtuin reaction, irrespective of whether you eat foods rich in sirtuin or not. Hence, include some few sirtuin foods to your diet: kale, walnuts, buckwheat, celery, are all great food. However, do not conclude that you cannot eat anything else. If you're determined about shedding weight, pay attention to lean protein, vegetables, and whole grains to reduce your total energy down.

You can discover your normal weight-loss calorie objective by locating your resting metabolic rate and then multiplying it by 1.3; let assume using exercise physiology and also sports nutritionist tips. Anything lesser than that, and you risk reducing your metabolism down.

Diet to activate sirtuins and promote health

It's apparently no accident that some of the individuals with long lifespan and healthiest populations in the world eat diets that are rich in these sirtuin-activating foods, examples are those in the Mediterranean and parts of Asia. The Mediterranean diet includes polyphenol-rich fruits, veggies, olive oil, including red wine. The Asian diet is rich in isoflavones present in soya beans and epigallactins from green tea.

Acquiring several of these health developing foods into your diet is proportionately easy. They can be included in many diets and even compound to make super-sirt meals!

Below are some great ideas you can get started with

Make use of olive oil for frying or roasting veggies or vegetables and salad dressings.

Ensure to own a jar of olives handy to snack on and include olives to salads or cooked meals. Tapenade usually makes a great topping for rye pieces of bread.

Exchange usual tea and coffee for green tea. Include a press of lemon for extra interest.

Miso alternatively can be used rather than stock cubes to flavor soups and stews. Milder light-colored miso may be used as a spread. Miso soup makes a great snack or soft meal if presented with salad or bread.

Include tofu or tempeh to stir-fries. Mix silken tofu into soups, immerse, and creamy desserts.

Put berries, blackcurrants to muesli, smoothies, and juices. Fresh yogurt, as well as fresh berries, ensure a healthy snack or dessert.

Take your greens. Cabbage and broccoli are outstanding support to any meal and can also be included in stir-fries, curries, stews, and casseroles.

Enrich up your life with turmeric and other spices. Don't restrict your input of seasonings to curries, include them to grains and vegetables.

Include cacao powder to smoothies and desserts too. Dredge cacao nibs on salads or include to trail mixes.

Apples are the ideal handy snack. Make sure you have one with you most times.

Buckwheat macaroni can be made as a tasty gluten complimentary option to wheat pasta, and buckwheat flour can also be made in baked products or to stiffer sauces. Buckwheat is also a great alternative that goes well with salads combined with roasted vegetables and toasted nuts.

Pros and Cons of Sirt food Diet

Pros:

- The 'sirt foods' apparently trigger the sirtuin in your body that is a type of protein that helps shield your cells from dying and contracting diseases, and also controlling your body metabolism.

- It's established on a research of 40 gym participants who each of them lost, on average 7lb in a week without losing muscle weight.

- You can eat normal amounts of dark chocolate and wine on a steady basis without you being affected.

- It consists of foods that are largely healthy and nourishing, such as blueberries, walnuts, and green tea.

- It is made to be effective for the long term and makes you healthy for life while also reducing the aging process.

Cons:

- For the first week, there is a calorie reduction that will eventually make most people lose weight, irrespective of what food is taken. This might occur as a result of the calorie restriction itself, which makes the participants shed weight. Also, for the first three days, you only take 1,000 calories daily, and the next four days requires to take up to 1,500 calories per day.

- Intensively reducing your calorie intake can be harmful if your body is not used to it and can make you sluggish.

- There is not enough proof that it follows through on its promises, most importantly the aspect of speeding up of your metabolism. Research on 40 people isn't much enough to say that it will eventually work as a healthy means to shed weight.

- You can only include foods on the sirt food list examples are 'sirt juices,' soy, green tea, and walnuts.

- In the conclusion of the above, there's less significance in having a variety of foods in your diet so as to look and feel good. For instance, eating fruit and vegetable every day provides enough minerals and vitamins in your meals at all times.

Chapter 5.   Positive Effects on our Body

They Fight Fat

When starting a diet, everybody expects to lose weight and feel great. However, you need to set the right expectations from the beginning. Also, you need to ask yourself this: Do you only want to lose plenty of weight in a short amount of time, or do you want to do this in a sustainable way?

The problem with most diets is that as soon as you quit them, you will get back to your unhealthy eating habits and you will recover the weight you lose. This has happened to many people after quitting their diet. The real challenge is to maintain your weight if you are satisfied with the weight loss so far.

This means that you have to stick to your diet, no matter what. The beauty of this diet is that it doesn't leave any food behind so it should be a lot easier to stick to it and enjoy it while you discover its benefits. When it comes to the fat-burning process, the most powerful sirtuin is SIRT1. As it turns out, bodies with a higher concentration of SIRT1 are leaner and have a more active metabolism. This was noticed in mice and can be easily applicable to humans. In other words, this specific sirtuin activates the skinny gene, capable of controlling your weight.

However, the benefits of SIRT1 don't stop there. It fights against PPAR-y (peroxisome proliferator-activated receptor-y), a group of nuclear receptor proteins responsible for the fat-gain process. These receptors simply trigger the genes required to synthesize and store fat. In order to prevent this from happening, PPAR-y must be stopped. Well, this is what SIRT1 does. It wipes out the production and storage of fat and speeds up your metabolism so your body can get rid of the excess fat. This can't be done without creating mitochondria (the energy factories from each of our cells). In other words, the more mitochondria you have (energy), the more fat you can burn, as it can allow you to engage in different physical fat-burning activities.

There are two kinds of fat storages: white adipose tissue (WAT) and brown adipose tissue (BAT). The first one is usually associated with weight gain fat, but the second one behaves differently, and it is even beneficial. This tissue is known for producing energy in the form of heat. Obviously, the WAT is the one you really need to work on, as this is the tissue that encourages fat accumulation, making us overweight or even obese. This is where sirtuins can perform a bit of magic, as they can make white adipose tissue to have the same properties as the brown one. This is what is called "the browning effect." In plain words, the fat from the WAT will be mobilized for disposal.

Sirtuins don't just encourage fat to disappear; it also has a very positive effect on insulin itself. As you probably know, weight gain is also associated with increased levels of insulin. SIRT1 can prove to be very helpful when it comes to lowering insulin resistance. Moreover, it encourages the release of thyroid hormones, so it has a crucial role in speeding up your metabolism and burning fat.

The sirtfood diet is also known for controlling your appetite, and I'm not talking about mind control encouraged by fasting; I'm referring to the "satiety hormone" known as leptin. The increase of leptin is making us satisfied as it decreases our hunger pangs. Make sense, right? Leptin is important as it is the hormone responsible for regulating your appetite. This is what should stop you from craving for more food, but in the case of obesity, leptin can't do its job properly. Why? Because of the hypothalamus, the brain doesn't sense that the body is well-fed, and it is constantly craving for more food, as somehow the brain believes the body is underfed. This situation is called leptin resistance.

Most overweight and obese people are addicted to carbs and processed food, the kind of food that can be named caloric bombs but have very poor nutritional value. The ingredients of a sirtfood diet can easily reverse leptin resistance. It makes sure that leptins signal your brain about the real level of nutrient intake. Moreover, people are really not experiencing hunger when trying this diet (unlike any fasting programs). Indeed, everything comes down to your brain, but when the right information reaches your brain (leptins), you have a much higher chance of controlling your appetite.

They Build Muscle Mass

When people mention that they want to lose weight, they are definitely referring to losing fat, not muscle. Fat is lighter than muscle, but we all want to have an optimal BMI, right? In the case of fasting, the growth hormone reaches incredibly high levels after 72 hours of pure fasting, so you can preserve and even increase your muscle mass through calorie deprivation.

However, the sirtfood diet is not rich in carbs; it is rich in sirtuins, a very healthy type of protein. The founders of this diet claim that you will lose seven pounds in seven days. With the sirtfood diet, you shouldn't experience any muscle loss. You might have this issue with radical diets, as you are losing fat and muscles at the same time. It is kind of a package deal. You will feel weak and lethargic. You will lack energy. Hence, you simply can't engage in any physical activities (that can at least preserve your muscle mass).

This meal plan is designed to save your muscles and only get rid of what you hate most: the unaesthetic fat tissue that makes you feel a lot heavy and not agile.

However, the food needs to create the right environment to build muscle mass or to preserve it, and this is what this diet is doing. After all, muscles are important for your mobility, and they prevent chronic diseases like osteoporosis or diabetes from happening. Believe it or not, but muscles can even have a psychological advantage, as they are known to fight against depression.

Fight Diseases

The modern-day eating habits and lifestyle encourages the accumulation of fats and toxins (fat tissue protects the toxins), as well as the increase of blood sugar and insulin level. This is where the trouble starts, from a simple pre-diabetes condition to more serious diseases (it can eventually lead to cancer). However, the antidote too many of these issues lies hidden within ourselves. As you already know, all bodies possess sirtuin genes, and activating them is crucial to burn fat and to build a stronger and leaner body.

As it turns out, the benefits of sirtuins activity extend way beyond the fat-burning process. Whether we like it or not, the lack of sirtuins can be associated with plenty of diseases and medical conditions. Naturally, activating sirtuins will have the opposite effect. For example, sirtuins can improve your heart health by protecting the muscle cells in your heart and improving the function of the heart muscle. But that's not all. Sirtuins can play a major role in improving the function of your arteries, controlling the cholesterol level, and preventing atherosclerosis.

By now, you are familiar with the effects of fasting and an LCHF diet on the insulin level, and you are probably wondering what sirtuins can do in this case. If you have diabetes, then you should know that activating sirtuins will make insulin work more effectively to do its job properly (which is regulating the blood sugar level). SIRT1 works perfectly with metformin (one of the most powerful antidiabetic drugs). As it turns out, pharmaceutical companies are adding sirtuin activators to metformin treatments. These studies were conducted on animals, and the results were simply amazing. It was noticed that an 83 percent reduction of the metformin dose is required to achieve the same effects.

Other diets or programs are bragging about their effects on neurodegenerative diseases, like Alzheimer's disease. Well, let's think about what sirtuins do! They send a message to the brain, helping it make the right decisions when it comes to appetite suppression. This involves enhancing the communication signals in the brain, improving the cognitive function, and lowering brain inflammation. Sirtuin activation stops the tau protein aggregation and amyloid β production, some of the most damaging things in the brains of Alzheimer's patients.

The benefits of sirtuins expand to bones as well, as they encourage the production of osteoblast cells (the ones responsible for strengthening your bones) and increase their survival. In other words, sirtuin activation is very important for overall bone health.

Now, we all know that the food we eat today can even lead to cancer, as we are literally eating small portions of poison. There are diets claiming that they represent the cure for cancer in an incipient form, but at the moment, we can't say this about sirtfoods, as there are still plenty of studies to be done on this topic. However, it is fair to say that people who eat mostly sirtfoods have the lowest cancer rates.

Losing weight is simply not enough nowadays, as the diet you have to follow needs to have plenty of health benefits as well; otherwise, you can't stick to it in the long run. Therefore, you need to see the bigger picture and not focus on losing a lot of pounds in a very short amount of time. Radical diets usually come with side effects, but if you find a meal plan that works for you in terms of weight loss and delivers plenty of health benefits, why not stick to it and make it your default diet? The less processed food you eat, the more chances you will have to experience the health benefits from your meal plan, so you don't have to see a doctor very often.

Natural ingredients have a lot of vitamins and minerals. They have a very high nutritional value. Coincidence or not, sirtuins can mostly be found in such ingredients (essentially fruits and veggies). Therefore, you will need to unleash these benefits on your body by consuming these amazing ingredients on a daily basis.

Anti-Aging Effect

SIRT1 can activate AMPK (and the other way around), so it can be considered one of the triggers of autophagy. There are a few ways to induce autophagy, and it obviously has a very positive effect on your health and overall lifespan. Just think of the cell as a car and autophagy is the skilled mechanic capable of fixing or replacing any broken parts in it. Obviously, the cell will have a longer life, and this extrapolates to your overall life. If your cells are functioning properly, like a Swiss mechanical clock, then you can expect increased longevity. You can't reverse aging, as there is no such cure for it, and autophagy is not "the fountain of youth." However, this process can significantly slow down aging and its effect. And the best part is that it can be activated by sirtuins, especially SIRT1.

Chapter 6.   Food for the Sirt Diet

Empowering Yourself with Sirt Foods

There are many uses and health benefits of Sirtfoods. Whether you are enjoying dark chocolate and wine or tofu and eggplant, you will find that you can enjoy these delicious ingredients in any meal or snack. We will be exploring the many health benefits these ingredients have to offer, along with some practical ways you can include them in your daily life. As you already know, Sirtfoods promote weight loss and weight management, so we will skip over these benefits and look toward other health benefits that they offer.

Buckwheat

Many people do not include buckwheat into their daily diets, but you should. Not only is it a great source of fiber, but it is also high in protein, and the carbohydrates will energize you when your calorie intake is limited. By adding in some buckwheat to your meals, you will help them stick with you longer, keeping you satisfied and energized longer than you otherwise would be. Another great bonus of buckwheat is that it is gluten-free, making it perfect for people with gluten intolerance or Celiac disease.

Dark Chocolate/Cocoa

One of the biggest benefits of dark chocolate is the role it plays in heart health. As many of the antioxidant sirtuins found within it are varieties especially helpful for heart health, you will find you can greatly reduce your risk of cardiovascular disease. A study published in 2015 found that when people eat chocolate daily, they have a reduced risk of heart disease and stroke. Another study found that when people eat dark chocolate five or more times a week, they reduce their risk of heart disease by fifty-seven percent.

Coffee

You may only think of coffee as a necessity to stay awake, or worse; you might even consider it an unhealthy addiction. However, just like tea has health benefits, so too does coffee. In a single cup of coffee, you can get plenty of vitamins B2, B3, B5, potassium, and manganese.

Kale

Kale is categorized as a calciferous vegetable, is a member of the cabbage family, and is considered one of the most nutritionally dense foods on earth. A single cup serving of ale contains large numbers of vitamins K, A, C, and B6, along with the mineral's manganese, copper, calcium, magnesium, and potassium. All this nutrition is packed in only thirty-three calories, making it a great choice to add to your daily diet.

Rocket Arugula

Arugula is unlike many other forms of lettuce, as it has a much stronger flavor that is distinct and peppery, adding a delicious flavor to several dishes. Even if a dish doesn't call for arugula, you can frequently add it in addition to or in lieu of other types of lettuce. Arugula is rich in potassium, calcium, vitamin C, vitamin K, vitamin A, and folate.

Capers

Frequently found in Mediterranean dishes, capers are immature flower buds that have been pickled. They have long been used throughout the world in ancient medicine, and now studies have proven that they are indeed great for health.

Extra Virgin Olive Oil

Olive oil is a notoriously heart-healthy source of fat, as it is largely made up of an incredible monounsaturated, known as oleic acid. This is the same type of fats that avocados are known for. This type of fat has been extensively studied and found to treat everything from skin conditions to cancer. Not only are these all great reasons to make the switch to extra virgin olive oil, but it is also resistant to heat, meaning it is useful in cooking.

Parsley

People usually only think of herbs as a source of flavor and not one for vitamins and minerals. But parsley will surprise you! It is high in vitamins C, K, A, folate, and potassium.

Matcha Green Tea

Green tea and matcha both come from the same type of tea plant. However, the way they are grown and prepared are different, leading to a more intense flavor and health benefits with matcha. When the leaves for matcha are grown, the farmers will cover the plants so that they don't receive direct sunlight for three to four weeks. When this is done, various nutrients in the leaf are increased, thus giving it the characteristic dark hue.

Celery

Celery might be incredibly low in calories, with only ten calories per stalk, but this crispy and fresh vegetables have many benefits aside from reducing your caloric intake. For instance, celery has approximately twenty-five different anti-inflammatory compounds in it, allowing it to greatly reduce inflammation all throughout the body, especially if enjoyed regularly.

Bird's Eye Chilies

A single tablespoon of chilies contains your daily requirements of vitamin C. This is not only great for your overall health and immune system, but it can also improve your hair and skin through its ability to strengthen collagen.

Soy

For a time, soy was demonized as potentially harmful food. Thankfully, science has shed light on the truth: that soy is a powerful superfood and sirtfood that has many health benefits. It is full of sirtuins, antioxidants, B vitamins, zinc, and iron. Not only is it nutritious, but studies have shown it to have numerous profound health benefits.

Turmeric

Turmeric has long been used both for food and medicine. In recent years, science has proven what those in India have long believed: turmeric has powerful health benefits. There are many reasons for these benefits, but one reason is the way it interacts with free radicals. Turmeric contains a powerful antioxidant, curcumin that can fight and neutralize free radicals to protect your cells. But it doesn't stop there.

Walnuts

Omega-3 fats, also found in fish such as salmon, is one of the most important fat to consume. If a person doesn't get enough omega 3, it can lead to chronic inflammation and a number of diseases. Thankfully, walnuts are a wonderful source of this important fat.

Blueberries

This little berry is low in calories but high in health benefits, such as its effects on the heart and the brain: two of the most vital organs. To help your heart, regular blueberry consumption can decrease LDL cholesterol. A single serving daily over a period of eight weeks was found to decrease LDL cholesterol by a shocking twenty-seven percent in one study. It can also reduce blood pressure by four to six percent over the same period. When combined, both effects greatly reduce a person's risk of heart disease.

Onion

Onions are another one of many sirtfoods that has a long history of being used in ancient medicine due to its profound health benefits. They have been used to treat several maladies such as heart disease, headaches, lung disorders, and mouth sores.

Strawberries

You can find many vitamins and minerals within strawberries, such as vitamins K and C, potassium, folate, magnesium, and manganese. These, combined with the polyphenols and other plant-based compounds, allow strawberries to boast a range of benefits. They have been found to lower LDL cholesterol, raise good HDL cholesterol, manage blood pressure, improve heart health, increase brain function, and improve skin and joint health, and much more.

Red Wine

We have conversed thoroughly throughout this book how red wine promotes heart health, but it can benefit other aspects of your well-being, as well. For instance, it can increase bone health, increase mental sharpness and response, and boost your gut health.

Cherries

Cherries are rich and full of antioxidants, sirtuins, vitamins, and minerals, all of which give them an abundance of health benefits. One such benefit is their ability to promote your workout recovery. While both sweet and tart cherries are beneficial, the tart variety is more effective for this. By drinking a little tart cherry juice, you can reduce inflammation, injury, and muscle pain brought about by your workouts. They can increase muscle recovery, allowing you to advance with fewer injuries and quicker healing physically. Some studies have also found that it can increase your exercise performance.

Cranberries

This tart little berry has long been known to help urinary health, which is especially helpful as one of the most commonplace types of bacterial infections is the UTI. Some people, especially women, struggle with these painful infections on a regular basis. But cranberries can help. They contain compounds that prevent dangerous bacteria, such as E. coli, from attaching to the lining of your urinary tract, and therefore preventing urinary tract infections before they can even begin. But, not only can they prevent the infections, but they can also help to treat them after the fact.

Red Cabbage

Higher in antioxidants and sirtuins than the more common green cabbage, red or purple cabbage still tastes the same. It is an incredibly versatile and low-calorie vegetable that you can add to a variety of dishes with ease.

Due to its ability to reduce chronic inflammation and lessen lesions in the stomach, red cabbage has many benefits for gut health. It is also high in fiber, which reduces constipation, increases nutrient absorption, lowers cholesterol, decreases hunger, and prevents blood sugar spikes. These benefits combined can prevent many common disorders centered on the digestive tract.

Eggplant

Also known as aubergine, eggplant has many health benefits from its combination of sirtuins, antioxidants, fiber, vitamins, and minerals. One of the many benefits this can impart is benefits to your heart health. In one study, it was found that both LDL cholesterol and blood triglycerides were reduced with regular consumption of eggplant juice in rabbits. Other studies have shown that eggplant can protect the heart against damage.

Cinnamon

What we know of as cinnamon is two different types of cinnamon. Known as "true cinnamon" is Ceylon cinnamon, but cassia cinnamon is what most people use today and refer to as cinnamon. While it used to be a precious commodity reserved for royalty, it is now something that nearly everyone can afford to keep in their spice cabinet. This is good news, considering its deep flavor and range of health benefits.

As you can see, sirtfoods are rich in nutrients and benefits, and we only went over a few benefits for each ingredient! There are many more benefits that we have not covered here that you can experience. By including sirtfoods into your daily diet, along with other components for a healthy and balanced diet, you can truly experience a range of health and weight loss benefits.

Chapter 7.   Diet Sirt and Physical Exercise

The expression of sirtuin in the muscle is affected by physical exercise that controls changes in the cellular antioxidant system, mitochondrial biogenesis, and oxidative metabolism.

Skeletal muscles are not only involved in force and movement but also engaged in endocrine activities by its ability to secrete cytokines and transcription factors into the bloodstream, thereby, controls the function of other organs. Furthermore, skeletal muscle is a metabolically active tissue that plays a vital role in maintaining the metabolism of the body. The skeletal muscle contains about 40% of the entire body weight. The insulin-stimulated uptake of glucose and the main energy-consuming lipid catabolism is mainly at this site. For the skeletal muscle, metabolic flexibility is essential to preserve physiological processes and metabolic homeostasis. It determines the ability to switch from glucose to lipid oxidation. Advances in the understanding of the molecular mechanisms underlying skeletal muscle activity are a therapeutic benefit. Sirtuins' roles have investigated in the skeletal muscle to their role in controlling glucose and lipid metabolism, insulin functions and sensitivity as well as function, and mitochondrial biogenesis.

Cellular metabolic stress results from physical exercise, which affects the sirtuins. The most studies sirtuins with this respect are SIRT1 and SIRT3, SIRT1 localized in the nucleus while SIRT3, in the mitochondria. SIRT3 expressed in type I muscle fiber. A research conducted showed that mouse skeletal muscle SIRT3 reacted to the six weeks voluntary exercise dynamically to coordinate the downstream molecular response (Palacios et al., 2009).

In summary, strenuous exercises activate SIRT1, which enhances biogenesis and mitochondrial oxidative capacity. Then, having several sessions of training will activate both SIRT1 and also SIRT3, which in turn enable ATP production as well as the mitochondrial antioxidant function.

Sirtuin activators boost your mitochondria's activity - the part of the biological cell which is responsible for the production of energy. In turn, mirrors the energy-boosting effects, which also occur due to exercise and fasting. The Sirt food diet starts a process called Adipogenesis, which prevents fat cells from duplicating – which should interest any potential dieter.

Tips for Success Diet

Fat burning, increasing muscles, and better cellular fitness—these are the guaranteed results of the Sirtfood diet.

Being healthy and losing weight is an everyday choice. You have to take those first baby steps and see how it can change you and your life.

If you want to reap the fantastic results of Sirtfoods, here are some suggested ways to jumpstart your diet:

Safety First

Before starting any particular diet or regimen, consult your healthcare provider, especially if you have an existing illness. It will ensure that this will not sabotage any medications that you might be taking or harm your health. Do not worry; the Sirtfood diet is reasonably safe.

Knowledge Is Power

This diet is still brand new, but there is always the right amount of information available and more upcoming since this diet is fast gaining popularity. You can also search the internet for recipes, food alternatives, nutrient content and more.

Follow the Guidelines

Sirtfood is guaranteed to bring results, if and only if you carefully follow the diet guide and suggested food.

Help Yourself

Aside from following what is allowed in the food program, you can start by eliminating processed and starchy food from your regular diet. Stop eating junk! It will fast track the result of Sirtfood Diet.

Start a Physical Activity

Sirtfood diet can indeed burn those fats and build muscle but also recommend that you start adding physical activities to your daily routine. A 30-minute walk a day would do wonders to your body and will also fast track the results. Also, there are many beautiful effects when exercising like preventing and combating health conditions, helping improve your mood, promoting better sleep, burning calories, giving you an energy boost and more.

Hit the Supermarket

The Sirtfood diet depends on certain foods. These foods have chosen because of their sirtuin-triggering ability. So if you do not follow the list, well, you won't see results.

Be Ready With the Initial Restrictions

Of course, if you want to see different results, you have to "sacrifice" a little to achieve the full benefits of the Sirtfood diet. But don't worry, the first three days are only the hardest ones for this diet since there will be calorie restrictions involved, but rest assured that it will become more comfortable each day. Although for others who tried this, the limitations set was not that hard for them, the reason is careful planning of meals. You will not go hungry with this diet if you choose wisely.

Plan Your Meals Ahead

Whatever diets you may be on, planning your meals is a big help. Not only will it reduce the stress from dieting, but you can also have the chance to weigh your choices and fill in your cupboard. You will be surprised that there are many filling dishes allowed with fewer calories and packed with sirtuins.

Involve a Diet Partner

This diet could also greatly benefit your family, partner or friends (not only for overweight individuals), plus it is easier when you have an accountability partner to remind you, share recipes or even cook dishes.

Document Your Progress

You can start by taking "before" pictures and take necessary body measurements. You could also keep a food diary so that you can watch your food intake. Observe the changes in your body with each week or phase. You can also have a set of goals to push you further to continue with the diet.

Be Kind to Yourself

Do not set too high expectations. Yes, some can quickly lose 7 pounds in a week, but remember that our bodies are not all the same; and of course, your level of commitment will also count. Other variables could be adding an exercise regimen in the diet plan, which could make the losing weight process faster.

Chapter 8.   Sirt Diet Phases

When the Sirt diet made headlines due to Pipa Middleton using it to lose weight before her wedding, it was only the beginning. Since then, Adele has achieved a stunning fifty-pound loss transformation, and everyday people, just like Adele, have achieved similar milestones all around the world. Whether a person is looking to lose ten, fifty, or more pounds, it is all possible when following the Sirt diet. But, not only is weight loss possible, there are a number of health benefits you may experience, as well! Many impartial and scientific studies have proven that sirtfoods can improve heart health, balance the immune system, decrease the risk of stroke, improve diabetic health, and much more! Here, we will be exploring the basic structure of the Sirtfood diet and what you can expect from it.

However, if you would like to go into more detail behind the science, possible health benefits, and step-by-step guides, then check out my book Sirt Diet. In that book, you will not only find the traditional Sirt diet approach, but you will also find my tailored approach that is perfect for slow and sustained weight loss if that is your goal. Whichever method you choose, you will find success.

The Sirt diet consists of two phases that last a total of three weeks. If you hope to lose more weight, then you can repeat these two phases in turn until you reach your goal weight. It's important that you do this, rather than lengthening the first phase, as the phases must be combined as intended for healthy weight loss. This is because the first phase, which lasts one week, reduces your kilocalorie intake, and the second phase is needed to balance this reduction. If you lengthen the first phase, you will not be offering your body the full nutrition it needs in the second phase. So, always remember, the first phase should never last longer than a week, and it should always be followed with the second phase. Now, let's examine these two phases.

During both phases of the diet, you will be drinking the signature Sirt green juice. The reason that this juice is important is that it offers you a number of sirtfoods in a concentrated form, activating your body's weight loss potential and boosting your health. This juice is an integral part of the diet and can't be skipped over. Thankfully, with just a few ingredients, you can easily make this juice in only a few minutes a day. I recommend making this juice first thing in the morning so that you always start your day by revving up your metabolism and boosting fat loss. While you will need multiple servings of green juice throughout the day, you can make it all in the morning and store what you will drink later in the day in the fridge, so that you only have to prepare it once a day. While it may be tempting to make all of your green juice at the beginning of the week, sadly, this is not an option. The reason for this is because science has found that after you make juice, every day that it is stored, it will lose an increasing number of nutrients. Due to this, you should never make your green juice more than one day in advance.

Phase One

The first phase of the Sirt diet lasts seven days. During this time, your kilocalories will be greatly reduced, and you will drink an increased amount of green juice a day to really push you to lose weight. This reduced kilocalorie intake is precisely controlled so that you stay healthy and still consume the nutrients your body requires. This phase is when you will lose the most weight, especially the first time you complete this phase as you will not only be losing fat, but also water weight.

In the first three days of this phase, you will be consuming one-thousand kilocalories per day. Days four through seven will include an increase to fifteen-hundred kilocalories a day. But, it is not all about restricting kilocalories, but also increasing nutrition and sirtfoods. Therefore, you will also be drinking three servings of green juice a day and, on average, eating two to three meals depending on how many kilocalories they contain.

While red wine is a classic sirtfood, it is only consumed after phase one. This is because the alcohol may hinder your weight loss if you drink it during the first phase, and due to your reduced kilocalorie intake, you could experience more intense side effects from drinking.

Phase Two

After the rapid weight loss in phase one, the second phase is designed to keep up your progress with weight maintenance. In this phase, your caloric intake is not reduced. You can freely consume; however, many kilocalories are recommended according to your BMI (body-mass index) and activity level. If you don't know your personal caloric recommendation, then you can easily find a BMI calculator online or ask your doctor.

You will continue to drink one serving of green juice daily, along with balanced healthy meals full of sirtfoods. The recipes in this book work for both phases of the diet, and you can simply eat; however, much is needed for your kilocalorie intake on a given day. But, you can also customize your favorite family recipes by including more sirtfoods in them. For instance, if your family loves pizza, then why not try adding some buckwheat to the crust and topping it with some onion, kale, and soy-based bacon replacement? By making pizza in this way, you can get four different types of sirtfoods. Of course, you shouldn't only consume sirtfoods. A healthy and balanced diet requires foods from all over the produce department, so make sure you eat a variety of fresh fruits and vegetables.

While the first phase lasts one week, the second phase lasts two weeks, or you can continue this phase indefinitely. Remember, if you want to increase your weight loss from the first phase, don't lengthen that phase. Instead, continue following both weeks of phase two, and then you can repeat phases one and two in turn. This will ensure you lose weight in a healthy and maintainable way.

Chapter 9.   The Sirtfood Diet Theory

The Sirtfood diet attempts to emulate the advantages of fasting diets, but without any of the drawbacks. You will learn about the theory of fasting diets and how the Sirtfood diet cleverly achieves the same effect, but without any of the actual fasting.

Many fasting diets have become popular in the past five years. The most well-known are the several variants of the intermittent fasting structure, such as the five-two diet. In the five-two diet, you fast during the weekend and eat normally during the working days of the week. These diets have proven and demonstrated effects on longevity, weight loss and overall health.

This is because these fasting diets activate the 'skinny gene' in our body. This gene causes the fat storage processes to shut down and for the body to enter a state of 'survival' mode, which in turn causes the body to burn fat.

Burning fat is what you might expect if you essentially start starving yourself, but another interesting effect of fasting is that your body switches from the replication of cells to the repair of cells.

Anytime cells in your body replicate there is a small chance of your DNA being damaged in the process. However, if your body repairs dying and older cells there is no risk of DNA damage, which is the reason why fasting is associated with lower prevalence of degenerative disease, such as Alzheimer's.

However, the problem with fasting diets, as the name implies, is that you have to fast. Fasting feels awful, especially when we are surrounded by other people having regular eating habits. It also puts some social spotlight on your own diet – explaining to your co-workers or your extended family why you are not eating on certain days is bound to generate incredulity and challenges to your diet regime.

Furthermore, even though fasting has numerous associated benefits, there are some downsides too. Fasting is associated with muscle loss, as the body doesn't discriminate between muscle mass and fat tissue when choosing cells to burn for energy.

Fasting also risks malnutrition, simply by not eating enough foods to get essential nutrients. This risk can be somewhat alleviated by taking vitamin supplements and eating nutrient rich foods but fasting can also slow and halt the digestive system altogether – preventing the absorption of supplements. These supplements also need dietary fat to be dissolved, which you might also lack if you were to implement a strict fasting method.

On top of this, fasting isn't appropriate for a huge range of people. Obviously, you don't want children to fast and potentially inhibit their growth. Likewise, the elderly, the ill and the pregnant are all just too vulnerable to the risks of fasting.

Additionally, there are several psychological detriments to fasting, despite commonly being associated with spiritual revelations. Fasting makes you irritable and causes you to feel slightly on edge – your body is telling you constantly that you need to forage for food, enacting physical processes that affect your mood and emotions.

This is why the authors of the Sirtfood diet sought a replacement for fasting diets. Fasting is clearly beneficial for our body, but it just isn't practical for society at large. This is where sirtuin activators and Sirtfoods come to the rescue.

Sirtuins were first discovered in 1984 in yeast molecules. Of course, once it became apparent that sirtuin activators affected a variety of factors, such as lifespan and metabolic activity, interest in these proteins blossomed.

Sirtuin activators boost your mitochondria's activity, the part of the biological cell which is responsible for the production of energy. This in turn mirrors the energy-boosting effects which also occur due to exercise and fasting. The sirtfood diet is thought to start a process called Adipogenesis, which prevents fat cells from duplicating – which should interest any potential dieter.

The interesting part is that the sirtuin activators actually influence your genetics. The notion of the 'genetic' lottery is embedded in the public consciousness, but genes are actually more changeable then you might think. You won't be able to change your eye color, or your height, but you can activate or de-activate certain genes based on environmental factors. This is called epigenetics and it is a fascinating field of study.

Sirtuin activators cause the SIR genes to activate, the before-mentioned 'skinny genes', which in turn increases the release of sirts. Sirts, or Silent Information Regulators also help regulate the circadian rhythm, which is your natural body clock and influences sleep patterns.

Sleep is important for many vital biological processes, including those that help regulate blood sugar (which is also important for losing weight). If you find yourself constantly stuck in a state of lag and brain fog, this may be caused by your circadian rhythm being out of sync, which is another way the sirtfood diet can help your body.

Additionally, sirts help contain free radicals. Free radicals are not as awesome as the sound – they are A.W.O.L particles in your body that damage your DNA and speed up the ageing process.

To summarize, the Sirtfood diet contains foods which are high in sirtuin activators. Sirtuin activators activate your SIR genes, or 'skinny genes' which enact beneficial metabolic processes. These processes, which involve molecules, called Sirts, causes your body to burn fat, repair bodily cells and combat free radicals.

Evidence

So, sirtfoods have been hailed as the next dietary wonder – but where is the cold, hard evidence? Well, the evidence for the sirtfood diet comes from multiple sources. To start with, Aidan Goggins and Glen Matten, the originators of the Sirtfood diet, performed their own trial at a privately-owned fitness center to test sirtfoods themselves.

At a fitness center called KX, in Chelsea, London the two authors of the sirtfood diet made a selection of their clientele eat a carefully monitored constructed sirtfood diet. What is particularly interesting about the study is that weight wasn't the only variable measured – the researchers also measured body composition and metabolic activity – they were searching for the holistic effect of the diet.

97.5% of people managed to stick to the first-three day fasting period, involving only 1000 calories. Generally speaking, this is a much higher rate of success than typical fasting diets, where many people have their willpower shattered in just the first few days.

Out of the 40 participants, 39 completed the study. In terms of overall fitness and weight, the individuals in the study were well distributed – 2 were officially obese, 15 fell into the overweight category whilst 22 had a regular body mass index. There were also 21 women and 18 men – a diet for both the genders! However, with that being said, being members of a fitness center the individuals in the study were more likely to exercise more than the standard population – a potential confounding factor.

Participants lost over 7lbs on average in the first week. Every participant experienced an improvement in body composition, even if their gains were not as dramatic as their peers.

There were also numerous reported psychological benefits, although these were not formally quantified. These improvements include an overall sense of feeling and looking better. As a side note, it was also claimed the 40 participants rarely felt hungry, even despite the calorie deficits imposed by the diet.

The most startling result from the sirtfood diet is that muscle mass after the 1-week diet period was either the same as before or showed slight improvements. Dieting law typically states that when losing fat, muscle is also lost, usually around 20-30% of the total weight loss, you should lose 2-3 lbs. of muscle for every 10 lbs. lost.

Of course, retaining muscle isn't just better from an overall fitness perspective, but also from an aesthetic view. A common fear, especially in men, is that if they lose weight is that they will look skinny, scrawny and unhealthy. Yet by the retaining the muscle you will gain that toned, slither look that is so fashionable in models.

Another important reason why retaining muscle mass is your resting energy expenditure. Your muscles require energy, even when you are not using them intensely. Owing to this, people who retain skeletal muscle burn more calories than people who don't, even if both people are sedentary. Basically, being muscular allows you to eat more calories and get away with it!

Muscle mass has also been associated with a general decrease in degenerative diseases as you age (such as diabetes and osteoporosis) as well as lower rates of mental health problems (such as depression and excessive anger).

Overall, the clinical trial performed at the KX fitness center not only supported the notion that the Sirtfood diet can aid weight loss and promote holistic body health, but it also led to the surprising finding that sirtfoods can retain muscle mass.

Blue Zones

The other evidence for the power of Sirtfoods comes from the 'blue zones'. The blue zones are small regions in the world where people miraculously live longer than everywhere else.

Perhaps most startlingly, you don't just see people live longer in blue zones; you still see them retain energy, vigor and overall health even in their advanced years. Most of us have the fear of becoming decrepit, immobile and overall miserable as we age.

Furthermore, we envision this as starting to occur in our forties and fifties, whilst becoming a fixed reality in our sixties, seventies and eighties. Yet in the blue zones, people not only live past 100 surprisingly regularly, but can walk, work and exercise just as well as those in the younger years. Likewise, they remain mentally slithe and don't suffer the cognitive deficits we typically associate with old age.

The blue zones include several areas of the Mediterranean, Japan, Italy and Costa Rica. What do these regions all have in common? They all eat a diet high in sirtfoods. The Mediterranean is famous for its healthy diet involving copious amounts of fish and olive oil. The Japanese savor matcha green tea, whilst the Costa Ricans traditionally indulge in cocoa, coffee and more.

This is the beauty of the sirtfood diet – it isn't trying to make your eating habits artificial and awkward. It is simply copying the healthiest practices that already exist around the world.

Chapter 10.   Breakfast Sirt Recipes

1. Soy Berry Smoothie

Preparation Time: 5 Minutes

Cooking Time: 0 Minute

Serving: 1

Ingredients:

1 cup fresh strawberries/blueberries (or frozen)

1 cup unsweetened vanilla soymilk

Directions:

Blend or blitz all the ingredients. Enjoy.

Nutrition:

Calories: 260 Cal

Carbs: 44 g

Sugar: 34 g

Fat: 4.5 g

2. Paleolicious smoothie bowl

Preparation Time: 5 Minutes

Cooking Time: 0 Minutes

Serving: 1

Ingredients:

1 piece Banana (frozen)

1 hand Spinach

1/2 pieces Mango

1/2 pieces Avocado

100 ml Almond milk

For garnish:

Mango1 / 2 pieces

Raspberries1 hand

Grated coconut1 tablespoon

Walnuts (roughly chopped) 1 tablespoon

Directions:

Put ingredients in a blender and mix to an even mass.

Put the mixture in a bowl and garnish with the remaining ingredients.

Of course, you can vary the garnish as you wish.

Nutrition:

Calories: 180 Cal

Carbs: 42 g

Sugar: 30 g

Fat: 31.5 g

3. Banana-Peanut Butter 'n Greens Smoothie

Preparation Time: 5 Minutes

Cooking Time: 0 Minutes

Servings: 1

Ingredients:

1 c. chopped and packed Romaine lettuce

1 frozen medium banana

1 tbsp. all-natural peanut butter

1 c. cold almond milk

Directions:

In a heavy-duty blender, add all ingredients.

Puree until smooth and creamy.

Serve and enjoy.

Nutrition:

Calories: 349.3 Cal

Fat: 9.7 g

Carbs: 57.4 g

Protein: 8.1 g

4. Fruity Tofu Smoothie

Preparation Time: 5 Minutes

Cooking Time: 0 Minutes

Servings: 2

Ingredients:

1 c. ice cold water

1 c. packed spinach

¼ c. frozen mango chunks

½ c. frozen pineapple chunks

1 tbsp. chia seeds

1 container silken tofu

1 frozen medium banana

Directions:

Add all ingredients in a blender until smooth and creamy.

Evenly divide into two glasses, serve and enjoy.

Nutrition:

Calories: 175 Cal

Fat: 3.7 g

Carbs: 33.3 g

Protein: 6.0 g

5. Green Vegetable Smoothie

Preparation Time: 5 Minutes

Cooking Time: 0 Minutes

Servings: 4

Ingredients:

1 c. cold water

½ c. strawberries

2 oz. baby spinach

1 lemon juice

1 tbsp. fresh mint

1 banana

½ c. blueberries

Directions:

Put the ingredients in a blender.

Nutrition:

Calories: 52 Cal

Fat: 2 g

Carbs: 12 g

Protein: 1 g

6. Creamy Oats, Greens & Blueberry Smoothie

Preparation Time: 4 Minutes

Cooking Time: 0 Minutes

Servings: 1

Ingredients:

1 c. cold fat-free milk

1 c. salad greens

½ c. fresh frozen blueberries

½ c. frozen cooked oatmeal

1 tbsp. sunflower seeds

Directions:

In a blender, put all ingredients until smooth and creamy.

Serve and enjoy.

Nutrition:

Calories: 280 Cal

Fat: 6.8 g

Carbs: 44.0 g

Protein: 14.0 g

Chapter 11.   Main Sirt Meals Recipes

7. Curry Chicken with Pumpkin Spaghetti

Preparation Time: 30 Minutes

Cooking Time: 2-4 Hours

Servings: 4

Ingredients:

500 g Chicken breast

2 teaspoons Chili powder

1 piece Onion

1 clove Garlic

2 teaspoons Ghee

3 tablespoon Curry powder

500 ml Coconut milk

200 g Pineapple

200 g Mango

1 piece Red pepper

1 piece Butternut squash

25 g Spring onion

25 g fresh coriander

Directions:

Cut the chicken (strips) and season with pepper, salt and chili powder. Then put the chicken in the slow cooker.

Finely chop the onion and garlic and lightly fry with 2 teaspoons of ghee. Then add the curry powder.

Deglaze with the coconut milk after a minute. Add the sauce to the slow cooker along with the pineapple, mango cubes, and chopped peppers and let it cook for 2 to 4 hours.

Cut the pumpkin into long pieces and make spaghetti out of it with a spiralizer.

Briefly fry the pumpkin spaghetti in the pan and spread the chicken curry on top.

Garnish with thinly sliced spring onions and chopped coriander.

Nutrition:

Calories: 140 Cal

Fat: 4 g

Fiber: 5 g

Carbs: 15 g

Protein: 15 g

8. French Style Chicken Thighs

Preparation Time: 20 Minutes

Cooking Time: 45 Minutes

Servings: 3

Ingredients:

700 g Chicken leg

1 tablespoon Olive oil

2 pieces Onion

4 pieces Carrot

2 cloves Garlic

8 stems Celery

25 g fresh rosemary

25 g Fresh thyme

25 g fresh parsley

Directions:

Season the chicken with olive oil, pepper and salt and rub it into the meat.

Roughly cut onions, carrots, garlic, and celery and add to the slow cooker. Sprinkle the chicken with a few sprigs of rosemary, thyme, and parsley on top. Cook for at least four hours.

Nutrition:

Calories: 140 Cal

Fat: 4 g

Fiber: 5 g

Carbs: 15 g

Protein: 15 g

9. Roast Beef with Grilled Vegetables

Preparation Time: 10 Minutes

Cooking Time: 30 Minutes

Servings: 3

Ingredients:

500 g Roast beef

1 clove Garlic (pressed)

1 teaspoon fresh rosemary

400 g Broccoli

200 g Carrot

400 g Zucchini

4 tablespoons Olive oil

Directions:

Rub the roast beef with freshly ground pepper, salt, garlic and rosemary.

Heat grill pan (high heat) and grill the roast beef for about 20 minutes.

Then wrap in aluminum foil and let it rest for a while.

Cut the roast beef into thin slices before serving.

Preheat the oven to 205 ° C. Put all the vegetables in a baking dish.

Drizzle the vegetables with olive oil and put curry powder and or chili flakes. Bake for 30 minutes.

Nutrition:

Calories: 140 Cal

Fat: 4 g

Fiber: 5 g

Carbs: 15 g

Protein: 15 g

10. Casserole with Spinach and Eggplant

Preparation Time: 20 Minutes

Cooking Time: 40 Minutes

Servings: 2

Ingredients:

1-piece Eggplant

2 pieces Onion

Olive oil 3 tablespoon

Spinach 450 g

Tomatoes 4 pieces

Egg 2 pieces

60 ml Almond milk

2 teaspoons Lemon juice

4 tablespoon Almond flour

Directions:

Preheat the oven to 200 ° C.

Cut the eggplants, onions, and tomatoes into slices and sprinkle salt on the eggplant slices.

Brush the eggplants and onions with olive oil and fry them in a grill pan.

Shrink the spinach in a large saucepan over moderate heat and drain in a sieve.

Put the vegetables in a greased baking dish: first the eggplant, then the spinach and then the onion and the tomato. Repeat this again.

Whisk eggs with almond milk, lemon juice, salt and pepper and pour over the vegetables.

Sprinkle almond flour over the dish and bake in the oven for 40 minutes.

Nutrition:

Calories: 140 Cal

Fat: 2 g

Fiber: 4 g

Carbs: 14 g

Protein: 12 g

11. Vegetarian Paleo Ratatouille:

Preparation Time: 10 Minutes

Cooking Time: 50 Minutes

Serving: 4

Ingredients:

200 g Tomato cubes

1/2 pieces Onion

2 cloves Garlic

1/4 teaspoon dried oregano

1 / 4 TL Chili flakes

2 tablespoon Olive oil

1-piece Eggplant

1-piece Zucchini

1-piece hot peppers

1 teaspoon dried thyme

Directions:

Preheat the oven (180 ° C) and lightly grease a round shape.

Finely chop the onion and garlic.

Mix the tomato cubes with garlic, onion, oregano and chili flakes, season with salt and pepper, and put on the bottom of the baking dish.

Use a mandolin, a cheese slicer or a sharp knife to cut the eggplant, zucchini and hot pepper into thin slices.

Put the vegetables in a bowl.

Drizzle the remaining olive oil on the vegetables and sprinkle with thyme, salt and pepper.

Cover the baking dish with a piece of parchment paper and bake in the oven for 45 to 55 minutes.

Nutrition:

Calories: 140 Cal

Fat: 2 g

Fiber: 4 g

Carbs: 14 g

Protein: 12 g

12. Vegan Thai Green Curry

Preparation Time: 10 Minutes

Cooking Time: 4 Hours

Servings: 2

Ingredients:

2 pieces green chilies

1 piece Onion

1 clove Garlic

1 teaspoon fresh ginger (grated)

25 g fresh coriander

1 teaspoon Ground caraway

1-piece Lime (juice)

1 teaspoon Coconut oil

500 ml Coconut milk

1-piece Zucchini

1-piece Broccoli

1-piece Red pepper

For the cauliflower rice:

1 teaspoon Coconut oil

1-piece Cauliflower

Directions:

For cauliflower rice, cut the cauliflower into florets and place in the food processor. Pulse briefly until rice has formed. Put aside.

Cut the green peppers, onions, garlic, fresh ginger and coriander into large pieces and combine with the caraway seeds and the juice of 1 lime in a food processor or blender and mix to an even paste.

Heat a pan (medium heat) with a teaspoon of coconut oil and gently fry the pasta. Deglaze with coconut milk and add to the slow cooker.

Cut the zucchini into pieces, the broccoli in florets, the peppers into cubes and put in the slow cooker. Simmer for 4 hours.

Briefly heat the cauliflower rice in 1 teaspoon of coconut oil, season with a little salt and pepper in a pan over medium heat.

Nutrition:

Calories: 140 Cal

Fat: 2 g

Fiber: 4 g

Carbs: 14 g

Protein: 12 g

□

13. Fruity Granola Bars

Preparation Time: 25 Minutes

Cooking Time: 30 Minutes

Serving: 24

Ingredients:

¾ cup packed brown sugar

½ cup honey

¼ cup of water

1 teaspoon salt

½ cup of cocoa butter

3 cups rolled oats

1 cup walnuts, chopped

1 cup ground buckwheat

¼ cup sesame seeds

½ cup dried strawberries or mixed fruits

½ cup raisins

½ cup Medjool dates, chopped

Directions:

In a large pan, combine sugar, cocoa butter, honey, water, and salt.

Stir in oats, walnuts, ground buckwheat, and sesame seeds. Cook, frequently stirring, for 15 minutes. Remove from heat and add dried fruits.

Pour into a large baking sheet lined with wax or parchment paper. Press firmly to create an even layer.

Score deeply into bars roughly 2" wide by 4" tall.

Allow cooling for 30 minutes before breaking or cutting along score lines. Store in an air tight container.

Nutrition:

Calories: 130 Cal

Fat: 4 g

Fiber: 5 g

Carbs: 15 g

Protein: 5 g

14. Cardamom Granola Bars

Preparation Time: 10 Minutes

Cooking Time: 1 Hour

Serving: 18

Ingredients:

2 cups rolled oats

½ cup raisins

½ cup walnuts, chopped and toasted

1 ½ teaspoons ground cardamom

6 tablespoons cocoa butter

1/3 cup packed brown sugar

3 tablespoons honey

Coconut oil, for greasing pan

Directions:

Preheat oven to 350 degrees F.

Grease the foil with coconut oil.

Mix the oats, raisins, walnuts and cardamom in a large bowl.

Heat the cocoa butter, brown sugar and honey in a saucepan until the butter melts and begins to bubble.

Bake for 30 minutes.

Allow cooling for 30 minutes. Lift the granola out of the pan and place on cutting board.

Nutrition:

Calories: 140 Cal

Fat: 4 g

Fiber: 6 g

Carbs: 10 g

Protein: 15 g

15. Coconut Brownie Bites

Preparation Time: 15 Minutes

Cooking Time: 30 Minutes – 2 Hours

Serving: 24-30

Ingredients:

2 ½ cups walnuts

¼ cup almonds

2 ½ cups Medjool dates

¼ cup unsweetened cocoa powder

1 teaspoon vanilla extract

¼ teaspoon of sea salt

¼ cup unsweetened desiccated or shredded coconut

Directions:

Roll into 1" balls.

Roll balls in coconut until well-covered and place on a wax paper-lined baking sheet.

Freeze for 30 minutes or refrigerate for up to 2 hours.

Nutrition:

Calories: 120 Cal

Fat: 3 g

Fiber: 5 g

Carbs: 15 g

Protein: 15 g

16. Tortilla Chips and Fresh Salsa

Preparation Time: 10 Minutes

Cooking Time: 10 Minutes

Serving: 4

Ingredients:

4 whole wheat flour tortillas

2 tablespoons extra virgin olive oil

4 Roma tomatoes, diced

1 small red onion, finely diced

1 Bird's Eye chili pepper, finely diced

2 teaspoons parsley, finely chopped

2 teaspoons cilantro, finely chopped

1 lime, juiced

Salt and pepper to taste

Directions:

Preheat oven to 350 degrees F.

Using a pastry brush, coat one side of each tortilla in olive oil.

With a sharp knife or pizza cutter, divide each tortilla into 8 wedges. Spread tortillas over a large baking sheet in a single layer. Use more than one baking sheet if necessary.

Bake for 8 – 10 minutes, flipping halfway through until both sides are golden brown and your chips are crispy.

While the chips are baking, combine tomatoes, red onion, chili pepper, parsley, cilantro and lime juice and mix well.

Serve salsa with the chips.

Nutrition:

Calories: 140 Cal

Fat: 4 g

Fiber: 5 g

Carbs: 15 g

Protein: 15 g

17. Garlic Baked Kale Chips

Preparation Time: 30 Minutes

Cooking Time: 5 Minutes

Serving: 2

Ingredients:

1 bunch kale leaves

½ tablespoon extra-virgin olive oil

1 teaspoon garlic powder

1/8 teaspoon cayenne powder

¼ teaspoon fine salt

Directions:

Preheat oven to 300 degrees F and cover a large baking sheet with parchment paper.

Remove the stems from your kale and tear up into large pieces.

Wash and spin the leaves until thoroughly dry, using a paper towel to pat dry if necessary.

Place kale leaves in a large bowl and massage the olive oil thoroughly into each leaf.

Combine garlic, cayenne and salt in a small bowl and mix well.

Sprinkle seasoning over kale and toss to distribute.

Spread kale in a single layer over the baking sheet.

Bake for 10 minutes, rotate the pan and bake for another 12-15 minutes more until the kale just begins to get crispy. The leaves will shrink and need to cool at least 5 minutes after being taken out of the oven to crisp properly.

Nutrition:

Calories: 150 Cal

Fat: 6 g

Fiber: 5 g

Carbs: 20 g

Protein: 20 g

18. Cauliflower Nachos

Preparation Time: 5 Minutes

Cooking Time: 20 - 25 Minutes

Serving: 4

Ingredients:

2 tablespoons extra virgin olive oil

½ teaspoon onion powder

½ teaspoon turmeric

½ teaspoon ground cumin

1 large head cauliflower

¾ cup shredded cheddar cheese

½ cup tomato, diced

¼ cup red bell pepper, diced

¼ cup red onion, diced

½ Bird's Eye chili pepper, finely diced

¼ cup parsley, finely diced

Pinch of salt

Directions:

Preheat oven to 400 degrees F.

Mix onion powder, cumin, turmeric and olive oil.

Core cauliflower and slice into ½" thick rounds.

Coat the cauliflower with the olive oil mixture and bake for 15 – 20 minutes.

Top with shredded cheese & bake for an additional 3 – 5 minutes, until cheese is melted.

In a bowl, combine tomatoes, bell pepper, onion, chili and parsley with a pinch of salt.

Top cooked cauliflower with salsa and serve.

Nutrition:

Calories: 150 Cal

Fat: 4 g

Fiber: 3 g

Carbs: 15 g

Protein: 17 g

Chapter 13.   Sirt Desserts Recipes

19. Pancakes with Apples and Blackcurrants

Preparation Time: 30 minutes

Cooking Time: 10 minutes

Servings: 4

Ingredients:

2 apples cut into small chunks

2 cups of quick cooking oats

1 cup flour of your choice

1 tsp. baking powder

2 tbsp. raw sugar, coconut sugar, or 2 tbsp. honey that is warm and easy to distribute

2 egg whites

1   ¼ cups of milk (or soy/rice/coconut)

2   tsp. extra virgin olive oil

A dash of salt

For the berry topping:

1 cup blackcurrants, washed and stalks removed

3 tbsp. water (may use less)

2 tbsp. sugar (see above for types)

Directions:

Place the ingredients for the topping in a small pot simmer, stirring frequently for about 10 minutes until it cooks down and the juices are released.

Take the dry ingredients and mix in a bowl. After, add the apples and the milk a bit at a time (you may not use it all), until it is a batter. Stiffly whisk the egg whites and then gently mix them into the pancake batter. Set aside in the refrigerator.

Pour a one quarter of the oil onto a flat pan or flat griddle, and when hot, pour some of the batter into it in a pancake shape. When the pancakes start to have golden brown edges and form air bubbles, they may be ready to be gently flipped.

Test to be sure the bottom can life away from the pan before actually flipping. Repeat for the next three pancakes. Top each pancake with the berries.

Nutrition:

Calories: 337 Cal

Fats: 6 g

20. Sirtfood Truffle Bites

Preparation Time: 1 Hour

Cooking Time: 0 Min

Servings: 15-20 pcs

Ingredients:

1   cup walnuts

¾ cup of Medjool dates, pitted

½ cup of dark chocolate broken into pieces; or cocoa nibs

2   heaping tablespoons of cacao powder

½ cup of dried coconut

1 tbsp. ground turmeric

1 tbsp. extra virgin olive oil or coconut oil (preferred)

1 tsp. vanilla extract, or a vanilla pod, scraped

1 dash of cayenne pepper

1   dash sea salt (up to 1/8 teaspoon)

2   tbsp. water if needed

Directions:

Pulse in a food processor the walnuts and chocolate until finely pulverized. Gently blend solid ingredients next and the vanilla. Make a dough. Make rolled balls out of the dough. Add water a few drops at a time only if I is necessary. Do not use too much water, or you will have to go and add more of the other ingredients to compensate. Refrigerate. Store for up to a week. Take them with you to work or when travelling for a quick pick-me-up as well as to quell a sweet tooth.

Nutrition:

Calories: 256 Cal

Fats: 15 g

21. Spicy Kale Chips

Preparation Time: 2 Hours 15 Minutes

Cooking Time: 15 Minutes

Servings: 1

Ingredients:

1 large head of curly kale, wash, dry and pulled from stem 1 tbsp. extra virgin olive oil

Minced parsley

Squeeze of lemon juice

Cayenne pepper (just a pinch)

Dash of soy sauce

Directions:

In a large bowl, rip the kale from the stem into palm sized pieces. Sprinkle the minced parsley, olive oil, soy sauce, a squeeze of the lemon juice and a very small pinch of the cayenne powder. Toss with a set if tongs or salad forks, and make sure to coat all of the leaves.

If you have a dehydrator, turn it on to 118 F, spread out the kale on a dehydrator sheet, and leave in there for about 2 hours.

If you are cooking them, place parchment paper on top of a cookie sheet, lay the bed of kale and separate it a bit to make sure the kale is evenly toasted. Cook for 10-15 minutes maximum at 250F.

Nutrition:

Calories: 345 Cal

Fats: 11 g

22. Sweet and Savory Guacamole

Preparation Time: 20 Minutes

Cooking Time: 0 Minutes

Servings: 2

Ingredients:

2 large avocados, pitted and scooped

2 Medjool dates, pitted and chopped into small pieces

½ cup cherry tomatoes cut into halves

5 sprigs of parsley, chopped

¼ cup of arugula, chopped

5 sticks of celery, washed, cut into sticks for dipping

Juice from ¼ lime

Dash of sea salt

Directions:

Mash the avocado in a bowl, sprinkle salt, and squeeze of the lime juice. Fold in the tomatoes, dates, herbs and greens. Scoop with celery sticks, and enjoy!

Nutrition:

Calories: 276 Cal

Fats: 14 g

23. Thai Nut Mix

Preparation Time: 30 Minutes

Cooking Time: 20 Minutes

Servings: 1

Ingredients:

½ cup walnuts

½ cup coconut flakes

½ tsp. soy sauce

1 tsp. honey

1 pinch of cayenne pepper

1   dash of lime juice

Directions:

Add the above ingredients to a bowl, toss the nuts to coat, and place on a baking sheet, lined with parchment paper. Cook at 250 F for 15-20 minutes, checking as not to burn, but lightly toasted.

Remove from oven. Cool first before eating.

Nutrition:

Calories: 322 Cal

Fats: 12 g

24. Berry Yogurt Freeze

Preparation Time: 1 Hour 30 Minutes

Cooking Time: 0 Minutes

Servings: 2

Ingredients:

2   cups plain yogurt (Greek, soy or coconut)

½ cup sliced strawberries

½ cup blackberries

1 tsp. honey (warmed) ½ tsp. chocolate powder

Directions:

Blend all of the above ingredients until creamy in a bowl. Place into two glass or in metal bowls that are freezer-safe, and put into the freezer for 1 hour, remove and thaw just slightly so that it is soft enough to eat with a spoon, makes two servings.

Nutrition:

Calories: 289 Cal

Fats: 16 g

25. Banana & Ginger Snap

Preparation Time: 30 Minutes

Cooking Time: 0 Minutes

Servings: 1

Ingredients:

2.5cm (1 inch) chunk of fresh ginger, peeled

1 banana

1 large carrot

1 apple, cored

½ stick of celery

¼ level teaspoon turmeric powder

Directions:

Place all the ingredients into a blender with just enough water to cover them. Process until smooth

Nutrition:

Calories: 324 g

Fats: 8 g

26. Chocolate, Strawberry & Coconut Crush

Preparation Time: 30 Minutes

Cooking Time: 0 Minutes

Servings: 1

Ingredients:

100mls (3½fl oz.) coconut milk

100g (3½oz) strawberries

1 banana

1 tablespoon 100% cocoa powder or cacao nibs

1 teaspoon matcha powder

Directions:

Toss all of the ingredients into a blender and process them to a creamy consistency. Add a little extra water if you need to thin it a little.

Nutrition:

Calories: 289 Cal

Fats: 16 g

27. Chocolate Berry Blend

Preparation Time: 30 Minutes

Cooking Time: 0 Minutes

Servings: 1

Ingredients:

50g (2oz) kale

50g (2oz) blueberries

50g (2oz) strawberries

1 banana

1 tablespoon 100% cocoa powder or cacao nibs

200mls (7fl oz.) unsweetened soya milk

Directions:

Place all of the ingredients into a blender with enough water to cover them and process until smooth.

Nutrition:

Calories: 256 Cal

Fats: 9 g

28. Mango & Rocket (Arugula) Smoothie

Preparation Time: 30 Minutes

Cooking Time: 0 Minutes

Servings: 1

Ingredients:

25g (1oz) fresh rocket (arugula)

150g (5oz) fresh mango, peeled, de-stoned and chopped

1 avocado, de-stoned and peeled

½ teaspoon matcha powder

Juice of 1 lime

Directions:

Place all of the ingredients into a blender with enough water to cover them and process until smooth. Add a few ice cubes and enjoy.

Nutrition:

Calories: 239 Cal

29. Summer Berry Smoothie

Preparation Time: 30 Minutes

Cooking Time: 0 Minutes

Servings: 1

Ingredients:

50g (2oz) blueberries

50g (2oz) strawberries

25g (1oz) blackcurrants

25g (1oz) red grapes

1 carrot, peeled

1 orange, peeled

Juice of 1 lime

Directions:

Place all of the ingredients into a blender and cover them with water. Blitz until smooth. You can also add some crushed ice and a mint leaf to garnish.

Nutrition:

Calories: 298 Cal

30. Buckwheat Pancakes with Strawberries and Chocolate Nut Butter

Preparation Time: 25 Minutes

Cooking Time: 25 Minutes

Servings: 8

Ingredients:

1.5 cups soy milk

1 cup buckwheat flour

1 large egg

1 tablespoon extra-virgin olive oil, for cooking

1 ½ cups strawberries, chopped

For the chocolate nut butter:

2/3 cup dark chocolate (at least 85%)

¼ cup milk

2 tablespoons double cream

1 tablespoon coconut oil

½ cup walnuts

Directions:

Place milk, flour and egg in a blender and blend until smooth. Transfer batter to measuring cup for easy pouring.

To make the chocolate nut butter: melt chocolate in a double-boiler, once melted, whisk in the milk, then the double cream and oil.

Pour into a blender with your walnuts and blend until smooth. For a saucier mix, add more milk or cream as desired.

To make the pancakes: warm a griddle to medium heat, adding small amount of oil as needed.

Pour batter onto griddle and cook until lightly browned on the bottom. Watch for air bubbles. You will know it's time to flip your pancake when the air bubbles pop.

 Flip your pancakes and cook until lightly browned on the other side. Repeat with remaining batter.

Top pancakes with strawberries and drizzle over with sauce, as desired.

Nutrition:

Calories: 278 Cal

31. Tropical Chocolate Delight

Preparation Time: 30 Minutes

Cooking Time: 0 Minutes

Servings: 1

Ingredients:

1 mango, peeled & de-stoned

75g (3oz) fresh pineapple, chopped

50g (2oz) kale

25g (1oz) rocket

1 tablespoon 100% cocoa powder or cacao nibs

150mls (5fl oz.) coconut milk

Directions:

Place all of the ingredients into a blender and blitz until smooth. You can add a little water if it seems too thick.

Nutrition:

Calories: 185 Cal

32. Blackcurrant and Raspberry Jelly

Preparation Time: 8 Minutes

Cooking Time: 7 Minutes

Servings: 2

Ingredients:

Raspberries – ½ cup (washed)

Blackcurrants – ½ cup (Washed and Stalks Removed)

Gelatin - 2 Leaves

Water - 300ml

Granulated Sugar - 2 Tablespoon

Directions:

Share the raspberries into two serving glasses or dishes. Soften the gelatin leaves by placing them in a bowl of cold water.

Place the blackcurrants in a small pan; add 100ml of water and the sugar. Allow to boil, and then simmer vigorously for five minutes before you put off the heat. Allow standing for two minutes.

Squeeze out any excess water from the leaves, and then add them to the saucepan. Stir together until fully dissolved, then add the rest of the water and stir. Pour the liquid into the serving glasses or dishes and place in the refrigerator to set, best to refrigerate overnight or a minimum of 3 to 4 hours.

Nutrition:

Calories: 354 Cal

33. Apple Pancakes with Blackcurrant Compote

Preparation Time: 20 Minutes

Cooking Time: 20 Minutes

Servings: 4

Ingredients:

Egg whites - 2

Plain flour – 1 cup

Porridge oats – ½ cup

Baking powder - 1 teaspoon

Pinch of salt

Caster sugar - 2 tablespoon

Apples – 2 (peeled, cored and chop into small pieces)

Light olive oil - 2 teaspoon

Semi-skimmed milk - 300ml

For the Compote

Blackcurrant– ½ cup (washed and stalks removed)

Water - 3 tablespoons

Caster sugar - 2 tablespoons

Directions:

The first step is to get your compote ready. Add the water, sugar, and blackcurrant into a small pan. Allow to simmer, and then cook for about 10 to 15 minutes.

Add the baking powder, salt, caster sugar, flour, and oats in a large bowl. Mix thoroughly. Add the apples, stir, and then whisk in the milk, a little at a time until you have a smooth consistency.

Whisk the egg whites to stiff peaks then add into the pancake batter. Move the batter into a jug.

Heat half teaspoon of oil in a non-stick fry pan over medium-high heat. Begin by pouring in approximately one-quarter of the batter. Cook on both sides until the batter turns golden brown. Remove the set and add the next batch until you have four pancakes.

Place the pancakes in a plate and drizzle the blackcurrant compote over them. Serve.

Nutrition:

Calories: 337 Cal

Chapter 14.   Vegetable Recipes

34. Sliced Potato Cake

Preparation Time: 15 Minutes

Cooking Time: 45 Minutes

Servings: 4

Ingredients:

2 lbs. potatoes

3/4 tsp. salt

3/4 tsp. pepper

1 tsp. dried Italian herbs

3 tbsp. olive oil

1 cup destroyed Parmesan cheddar

Directions:

Wash and strip the potatoes. Cut them into meagre cuts (ideally with a mandolin). Spot the vegetables into an enormous blending bowl. Include the oil, salt, pepper, and Italian herbs. Utilizing your hands, blend tenderly, ensuring the entirety of the cuts is prepared. Include the Parmesan and blend delicately. Spot material paper onto an enormous heating sheet and spot a 10" Spring form Pan without the base on top. Include the potato blend inside and spread it pleasantly. Evacuate the spring form Pan Ring. Prepare in a preheated stove at 375°F for around 50-55 minutes, until the potatoes look brilliant dark-colored and are cooked through.

Nutrition:

Calories: 119 Cal

Fat: 40 g

35. White Beans with Garlic, Sage and Tomatoes

Preparation Time: 15 Minutes

Cooking Time: 2 Hours

Servings: 3

Ingredients:

1 cup dried cannellini beans

1/4 cup olive oil

Four cloves garlic, minced around 2 tbsp.

Four new sage leaves, cleaved around 1 tbsp.

1/4 cup dry white wine

1 28 Oz can San Maranon tomatoes depleted

Genuine salt and crisply ground dark pepper to taste

Directions:

Spread the beans with water in a huge pot and let drench medium-term. Channel beans and re-load up with a new pool in the same Pan. Heat to the boiling point and cook for 1/2 to 2 hours, or until beans are delicate. Channels beans, saving around 1 cup of fluid. In a large skillet over medium warmth, warm the olive oil. Include the garlic and sage and cook until daintily brilliant, around 2 minutes. Include the wine and cook until almost dissipated about 3 minutes. Include the beans and the press the tomatoes into the seeds with your hands. Season with a sound touch of salt and pepper. Stew for 15 minutes, including saved fluid if getting dry. Move to a serving bowl and serve without a moment's delay, or serve at room temperature.

Nutrition:

Calories: 112 Cal

Fat: 40 g

36. Eggs and Broccoli Salad with Yogurt Dressing

Preparation Time: 40 Minutes

Cooking Time: 40 Minutes

Servings: 2

Ingredients:

3 eggs

1 pound of broccoli

3 small sun-dried tomatoes

1 tbsp. walnuts

¾ cup of yogurt

Black pepper to taste

1 tsp. mustard

1 tsp. extra virgin olive oil

1 garlic clove

5 brown champignon mushrooms

Directions:

Put eggs in cold water and bring to a boil. Leave them in the boiling water for 8 to 10 minutes, until they are hard-boiled.

While the eggs cook, wash and cut the broccolis in thin slices

Cut the tomatoes in thin slices, as well.

Bring a pot of water to a boil and the let the broccoli cook for 5 to 7 minutes, for the last 3 minutes of cooking add the tomatoes too.

Toast without fats the walnuts

Prepare the dressing, mixing well together the yogurt, pepper, mustard, and oil.

Wash and cut the champignons in thin slices

Mix all the vegetables with the dressing in a medium bowl. Let rest for 10 minutes.

Cut the hard-boiled eggs in quarters, add to the salad, and top it with the toasted walnuts

Nutrition:

Calories: 2 26 Cal

Fat: 31 g

37. Tuscan Bean Casserole

Preparation Time: 30 Minutes

Cooking Time: 30 Minutes

Servings: 1

Ingredients:

1 tablespoon extra-virgin olive oil

1 /3 cup (50g) red onion, finely chopped

1 /4 cup (30g) carrot, peeled and finely chopped

1 /3 cup (30g) celery, trimmed and finely chopped

2 garlic cloves, finely chopped

1 /2 Thai chili, finely chopped (optional)

1 teaspoon herbes de Provence

7 /8 cup (200ml) vegetable stock

1 x 14-ounce can (400g) chopped Italian tomatoes

1 teaspoon tomato purée

3 /4 cup (130g) canned mixed beans (drained weight)

3 /4 cup (50g) kale, roughly chopped

1 tablespoon roughly chopped parsley

1 /4 cup (40g) buckwheat

Directions:

Place the oil in a medium saucepan over low to medium heat and gently fry the onion, carrot, celery, garlic, chili (if using), and herbs, until the onion is soft but not browned.

Add the stock, tomatoes, and tomato purée and bring to a boil.

Add the beans and simmer for 30 minutes. Add the kale and cook for another 5 to 10 minutes, until tender, then add the parsley.

Meanwhile, cook the buckwheat according to the package instructions, drain, and then serve with the stew.

38. Baked Tofu with Harissa on Spiced Cauliflower Couscous

Preparation Time: 70 Minutes

Cooking Time: 70 Minutes

Servings: 1

Ingredients:

3 /8 cup (60g) red bell pepper

1 Thai chili, halved

2 garlic cloves

About 1 tablespoon extra-virgin olive oil

Pinch of ground cumin

Pinch of ground coriander

Juice of 1 /4 lemon

7 ounces (200g) firm tofu

1 3 /4 cups (200g) cauliflower, roughly chopped

1 /4 cup (40g) red onion, finely chopped

1 teaspoon finely chopped fresh ginger

2 teaspoons ground turmeric

1/2 cup (30g) sun-dried tomatoes, finely chopped

1/2 cup (20g) parsley, chopped

Directions:

Heat the oven to 400°F (200°C).

To make the harissa, slice the red pepper lengthwise around the core so you have nice at slices, remove any seeds, then place in a roasting pan with the chili and one of the garlic cloves.

Toss with a little oil and the dried cumin and coriander and roast in the oven for 15 to 20 minutes until the peppers are soft but not too browned. (Leave the oven on at this setting.)

Cool, then blend in a food processor with the lemon juice until smooth.

Slice the tofu lengthways and then cut each half diagonally into triangles.

Place in a small nonstick roasting pan or one lined with parchment paper, cover with the harissa, and roast in the oven for 20 minutes—the tofu should have absorbed the marinade and turned dark red.

To make the "couscous," place the raw cauliflower in a food processor.

Pulse in 2-second bursts to finely chop the cauliflower until it resembles couscous. Alternatively, you can just use a knife and chop it very finely.

Nutrition:

Calories: 227 Cal

Fat: 13 g

39. Spinach and Kale Stir Fry

Preparation Time: 15 Minutes

Cooking Time: 15 Minutes

Servings: 4

Ingredients:

2 chopped shallots

1 cup no-salt-added and chopped canned tomatoes

2 cup baby spinach

2 minced garlic cloves

5 cup torn kale

1 tbsp. extra virgin olive oil

Directions:

Heat up a pan with the oil over medium-high heat

Add the shallots, stir and sauté for 5 minutes.

Add the spinach, kale, and the other ingredients, toss, cook for 10 minutes more.

Divide between plates and serve.

Nutrition:

Calories: 141 Cal

Fat: 28 g

40. Aromatic Red Endives

Preparation Time: 30 Minutes

Cooking Time: 30 Minutes

Servings: 4

Ingredients:

2 tbsp. extra virgin olive oil

1 tsp. dried rosemary

2 halved endives

¼ tsp. black pepper

½ tsp. turmeric powder

Directions:

In a baking pan, combine the endives with the oil and the other ingredients, toss gently.

Insert in the oven and bake at 400 0F for 20 minutes.

Divide between plates and serve.

Nutrition:

Calories: 102 Cal

Fat: 38 g

Conclusion

Thank you for making it to the end. Indeed, 6 out of every 10 Americans are currently struggling to live their lives through the pain and discomfort of disease, but these statistics don't have to keep declining. You now have enough knowledge to make lifestyle changes that will protect you from being on the wrong end of these statistics.

Despite the incredible advances that science has made in the fields of health, the body, and medicine, our world is getting sicker by the day. I believe that part of this reason is that this knowledge is being passed around only by an elite few doctors, researchers, and dieticians. The more you know about your own body, the more power you can control to protect your health.

It doesn't matter where your health is right now. What matters is what you're going to do about it from now on. You know you need to change and, hopefully, you now have a good foundation in some simple, effective, and relatively enjoyable ways you can change your health for the better.

This book was written to be much more than just another diet book. The goal was to spark excitement and interest in your heart about your health. Too many of us go through our lives, assuming that we should not be held responsible for our health – that is the realm of doctors and professional healers.

But the more you can learn about how your body operates, the better equipped you will be to take control of your health, rather than waiting for it to deteriorate to the point where you need a doctor's intervention.

The human body is a remarkable machine. It is designed with a more advanced natural defense system than current medical science even fully understands. However, the amount we do know tells us that for these natural defenses to protect us from disease effectively, they need two things: energy and nutrition.

Those components also need to be well balanced, as too much or too little energy can throw the entire system off balance.

The 21st century has given us an incredible bounty of food, so we have all the energy and nutrition available to us easily, without being forced to hunt it down for ourselves as our ancestors did.

Unfortunately, we also have an abundance of new foods available to us. Foods that over-deliver on the first requirement, energy, and under-deliver on the second requirement, nutrition. Knowing this, we can work towards finding the right balance once again.

With every additional nutrient-dense sirtuin-activating food source you consume, you are proactively working towards rebalancing those scales.

The Sirtfood Diet is not a temporary or quick fix, but it is a lifestyle that you can adapt to prioritize your health for the rest of your life.

Temporary weight loss followed by sustained weight gain is the way of calorie restricting, time-bound diets. They're unpleasant to follow, often require a lot of math and calculations, and are not serving you.

Diets that are rich in delicious and health-supporting nutrition help your body optimize itself. The Sirtfood Diet isn't about restricting anything in your life. It's focused on all the good things you can add to feel great, look fantastic, and become the healthiest, best version of yourself at any age or stage in your life.

This book did not set out to give you an official diet blueprint to follow, planning out your every bite for you. Instead, the goal was to help you understand the value of the foods you choose to eat so that you can learn how to make these choices automatically and with full confidence.

Of course, it always helps to have a selection of choices to choose from, so now that you're ready to start this Sirtfood Diet for yourself, you can flip the next few pages to find Appendix 1 and 2, a combined list of 120 food choices that are sirtuin-activating and rich in polyphenols.

You're ready to start living your best life, and you deserve to feel healthy, energetic, and beautiful. To help you make these conditions of a great life a reality for you, the Sirtfood Diet is the last diet you will ever need.

Congratulations and Bon Appetite!